A
short &
informative guide
to becoming a

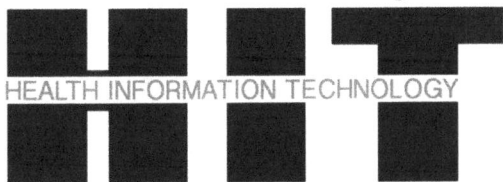

HIT

HEALTH INFORMATION TECHNOLOGY

STUDENT

KELLI LEWIS

KELLI LEWIS

Published by

M&L Media Publishing

ISBN:069227653X
ISBN-13:9780692276532

DEDICATION

To my Mother, for believing in me and your
continued love and support.

To my Brother, for your love and
encouragement.

To my Ancestors, whose shoulders I stand on.

KELLI LEWIS

PREFACE

by Kelli Lewis, MSHI, RHIA

Why I wrote this book?..... The profession of Health Information Management has been around for over eighty years however, many people are not aware of this rewarding profession and the many career options it offers. Also, many people are not aware that even though they may not want to have direct patient contact, they still have a career in a allied health profession that makes a difference in patients lives.

I wanted to write this book to introduce readers to the Health Information Technology profession, to help new and aspiring students discover a successful career in Health Information Technology, and inspire individuals looking for a career change.

It is my hope that this book will provide answers and information to students who are trying to decide on a degree to major in, individuals who are interested in learning more about the profession, and to assist teachers. This book provides readers with the rich history of the profession, career options, and how to advance your career. After reading this book it is my belief that you will discover a new career and have an appreciation for this great profession.

CONTENTS

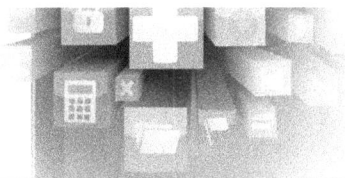

INTRODUCTION

Are you still pondering what to major in? Maybe you can't find the right job, have lost your job, or perhaps, you are looking for more meaningful work. Have you ever thought about having a career in healthcare but prefer not to deal directly with patients? Consider majoring in Health Information Technology and becoming a Health Information Technician. Health Information Technology is different than many other allied health jobs in that it requires computer proficiency rather than direct, hands on patient care. Employment of health information technicians is expected to increase by 21% from 2010 to 2020, faster than the average for all occupations. Projections indicate that career opportunities in health information technology are tremendous. The U.S. Bureau of Labor Statistics predicts that job opportunities for health information technicians will be highly favorable in the coming years.

Ready for a career change or maybe what your first career will be?

This book in a short period of time gives the reader an overview of what health information technology is, career options, and things students should do while enrolled in a health information technology program. This book will take you on a journey hopefully leading to a destination of a fulfilling career.

MAXIMIZING YOUR

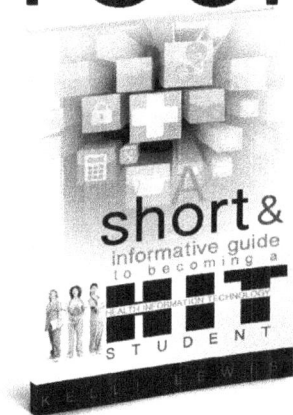

DISCOVERY EXPERIENCE

1. **Read the table of contents**. It will introduce you to the contents of the book and its chapters.
2. **Learn about the profession of health information technology in chapter 1**. Pay special attention to how long the profession of health information management has been in existence.
3. **Gain understanding about the employment options available to health information technicians in chapter 2**. Take time to read the descriptions of the jobs listed and earning potential.
4. **Review the education options available to you by reading chapter 3.** This chapter will explore the degrees you can earn and various education delivery formats.
5. **Gain insight into how to survive your first year, as a Health Information Technology student in chapter 4.** In this chapter you will learn about things you should be doing and participating in to make the most out of your first year as a health information technology student.
6. **Pinpoint ways in which you should be preparing for certification in chapter**

5. This chapter will provide you with suggestions and study tips for preparing for your certification exam.

7. **Put your career to work in chapter 6.** In this chapter you will be given tips to use in landing your first job as a health information technician.

8. **You have landed your first job but, don't let your learning stop in chapter 7.** In this chapter we will discuss the importance of continuing your education to maintain your certification(s) and expand your expertise.

Finally, we will explore additional resources that you can use to expand your knowledge about the health information technology profession. Make sure you peruse through each chapter carefully so you don't miss a single piece of advice. By following the suggestions you will get answers to some of the most important questions and clearly define your career choice. Don't wait any longer. Start your journey to learning more about the profession of health information technology.

KELLI LEWIS

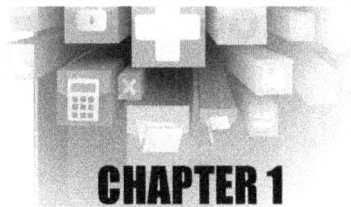

CHAPTER 1
HISTORY OF THE PROFESSION

The premier professional association worldwide
for health information technicians is the
American Health Information Management
Association (AHIMA). AHIMA traces its
history back to 1928. The health information
management profession evolved from the need
for accurate and complete records regarding the
care and treatment of patients as one means to
improve and standardize healthcare. The
American College of Surgeon's (ACS)
standardization program lead the efforts to
organize and educate a group of people who
could assist hospitals in meeting the
informational needs of accrediting bodies and
medical educators. Hospital medical record
departments were forming and a knowledgeable
workforce was needed to implement and

manage the collection, storage, and retrieval of patient data and records.

In 1928, the ACS invited medical record workers from the United States and Canada to attend their meeting which resulted in the medical record workers organizing to form the Association of Record Librarians of North American (ARLNA). The first meeting of the ARLNA was held in Chicago, the following year members adopted a constitution, bylaws, and formed a committee to develop a course of study for medical record librarians. The Canadian members of the association eventually broke away and formed their own association in 1944. The curriculum for medical record librarians was finalized in 1932 and the first academic programs were approved in 1934. Over the years the Association has had name changes to accommodate the evolution of the profession. Today the association is known as American Health Information Management Association (AHIMA).

AHIMA serves 52 affiliated components state associations, and more than 71,000 members, it is recognized as the leading source of "HIM knowledge". In addition, to providing resources AHIMA actively advocates for the health information management profession, serves as a thought leader in the world of health information management and is one of the four parties responsible for ICD-10 coding guidelines. For additional information please visit the American Health Information Management Association website at *www.ahima.org*

What is Health Information Technology?

Health Information Technology incorporates science, business, management, law, and technology. According to the American Health Information Management Association health information professionals care for patients by caring for their medical data. My state association the Florida Health Information Management Association states whenever healthcare is provided, a medical record must be created, reviewed, and stored. Health information technicians ensure a patients' health information is organized and that the information is complete, accurate, and protected in both paper and electronic systems. While some tasks may vary by employer and specialty health information technicians typically review patients records for timeliness, completeness, accuracy, and appropriateness of data, organize and maintain data for clinical databases and registries, track patient outcomes for quality assessment, use classification software to assign clinical codes for reimbursement and data analysis, electronically record data for collection, storage, analysis, retrieval, and reporting, and protect patient health information for confidentiality authorized access for treatment, and data security. (Occupational Outlook Handbook, 2014)

Health information technicians do not provide direct patient care however; they do work regularly with doctors, nurses and other healthcare professionals. Health information technicians meet with these healthcare professionals to clarify diagnoses or to get additional information to make sure that records are complete and accurate. (Occupational Outlook Handbook, 2014)

With an aging population and population growth the demand for health services is expected to increase thus creating more medical information that must be collected, organized, and analyzed. With many facilities transitioning from paper to electronic health records (EHR) it has increased the job opportunities available to health information technician professionals. Federal legislation is providing incentives for physicians' office and hospitals to implement electronic health records systems into their practice.

Health information technicians will need to be familiar with electronic health record software, follow electronic health record security and privacy practices, and analyze electronic data to improve healthcare information as more healthcare providers and hospitals adopt electronic health record systems.

Skills and qualities needed to be a health information technician:

- Computer skills- much of the jobs that health information technicians do is computer related. Basic computer skills such as typing, file retrieval, and data entry are essential.
- Analytical skills- health information technicians must be able to understand and follow medical record diagnoses to decide the best codes to use.
- Detailed oriented- health information technicians must ensure the integrity of

data, such as making sure information is complete and accurate.

- Personal interaction skills- health information technicians must be able to interact with a variety of people such as administrators, doctors, nurses, allied health professionals, and patients.

KELLI'S
CAREER
CHRONICLES

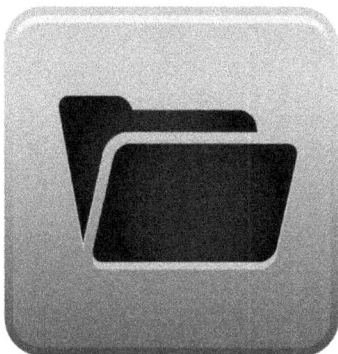

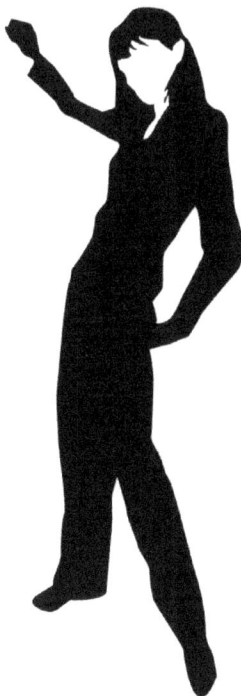

When I went to college I had no idea there was a profession called health information management. I knew I wanted to be an allied health professional but, I wasn't sure exactly which field I wanted to major in so as a freshman in college I declared health science as my major. During my first year of college I took a Medical Terminology course in which the professor happened to be a Health

Information Management professional. The professor who I could tell had a passion for her profession, told me about the field of health information management and the many exciting career choices that a person could have with a bachelor's degree. After learning about the career options and finding out that it would combine my love of science and technology that was enough for me I changed my major to health information management what a great career choice it has been!

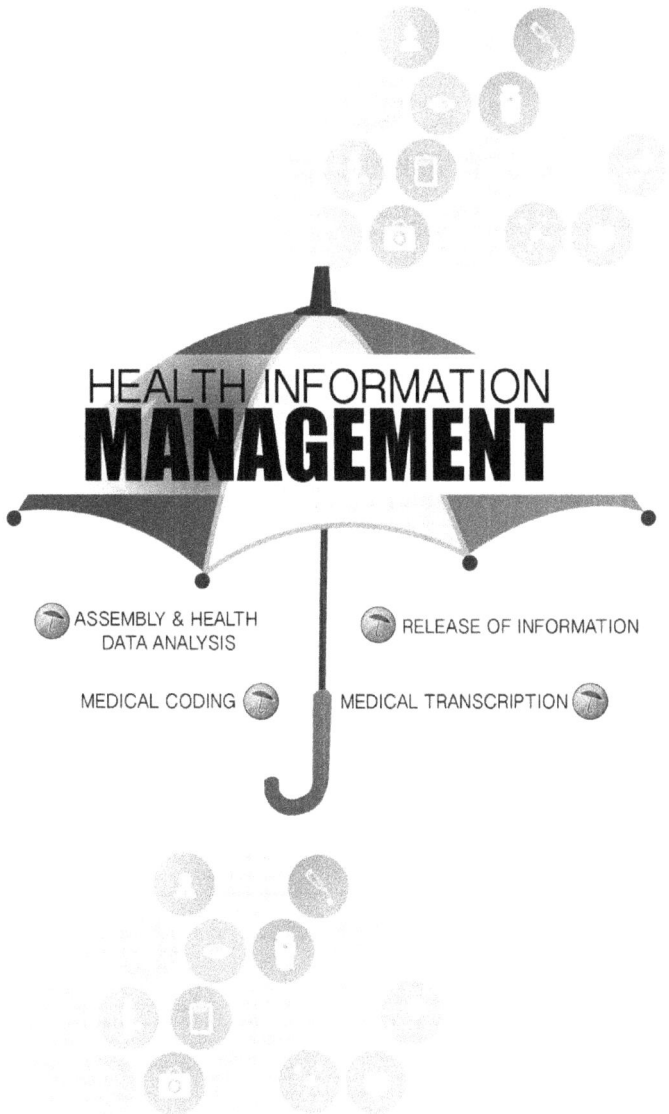

HEALTH INFORMATION
MANAGEMENT

ASSEMBLY & HEALTH
DATA ANALYSIS

RELEASE OF INFORMATION

MEDICAL CODING

MEDICAL TRANSCRIPTION

KELLI'S
CALL TO ACTION

What interests you most about the HIT profession? Why?

_____
_____
_____
_____
_____
_____
_____
_____
_____
_____
_____
_____
_____
_____
_____

Which skill and/or quality mentioned will you need to further develop to become a successful HIT professional?

_____

How do you plan to further develop this?

_____

_____

_____

_____

_____

_____

_____

_____

_____

_____

_____

_____

_____

_____

_____

_____

_____

_____

Chapter Highlights

_____

_____

_____

_____

_____

_____

_____

_____

_____

_____

_____

_____

_____

_____

_____

_____

_____

_____

_____

_____

_____

_____

_____

_____

_____

_____

_____

Action Items

- _____

- _____

- _____

- _____

- _____

- _____

- _____

- _____

- _____

- _____

- _____

- _____

Notes

_____
_____
_____
_____
_____
_____
_____
_____
_____
_____
_____
_____
_____
_____
_____
_____
_____
_____
_____
_____
_____
_____
_____
_____
_____
_____
_____
_____

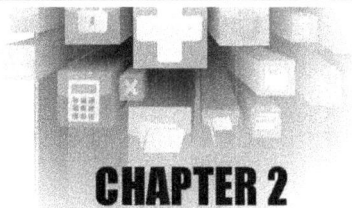

CHAPTER 2
EMPLOYMENT OPPORTUNITIES

Wherever health information is maintained there is an employment opportunity for health information technicians. Employment of health information technicians is expected to increase by 21% from 2010 to 2020, faster than the average for all occupations. Projections indicate that career opportunities in health information technology are tremendous. The Bureau of Labor Statistics attributes this employment growth to the use of electronic health records and an aging baby boomer population that will utilize healthcare services. For additional information please refer to the Occupational Outlook Handbook, 2014.

Employment opportunities are available in different types of health care settings. Most health information technicians work in hospitals. Others work in nursing care facilities or for government entities. Some settings outside of the hospital setting that health information technicians may work include correctional facilities, insurance companies, software vendors, veterinary medicine. Technicians typically work at a desk and spend most of their time at their computer.

Health Information Technology Jobs

Jobs that health information technicians can have include release of information specialist, medical record coder, cancer registry, and health data analyst.

Release of Information Specialist- process release of information requests in a timely manner according to state and federal laws. The release of information specialist is responsible for maintaining the patient's privacy and maintaining confidentiality.

Medical Coder- Assigns codes (numbers) to the diagnosis and procedures that the patient has had based on the documentation provided in the patients record.

Cancer Registrar- Responsible for reporting cancer statistics to the government and healthcare agencies. Cancer registrars collect and analyze the medical information of cancer patients. The information the cancer registrars collect and report is essential for researchers and advancements in treatments.

Health Data Analyst- Analyze the patient medical record for any deficiencies and incompletes or delinquent records.

The following positions release of information specialist, medical coder, cancer registrar, and health data analyst, require at least an associate degree. However, some facilities will hire medical coders without an associate degree and only certification. Cancer registrar and medical coding are considered specialties. Some health information technicians specialize in being a cancer registrar or medical coder which in addition to formal education requires certification for employment. See chapter 5 for types of certifications health information technicians may have.

Salary:

The median annual wage for health information technicians was $34,160/ 16.42 per hour in May 2012. The lowest 10 percent earned less than $22,250 and the top 10 percent earned more than 56,200. Most health information technicians work full time in healthcare facilities that are always open and have the option of working evenings or overnight if they choose. For additional information please see the Occupational Outlook Handbook, 2014. Salaries vary by the size of the organization and the region of the country where one resides in. The more education and credentials you have the higher your earning potential.

KELLI'S
CAREER
CHRONICLES

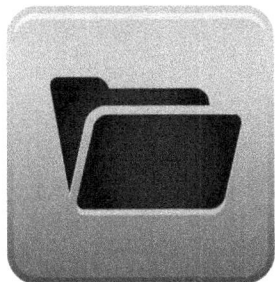

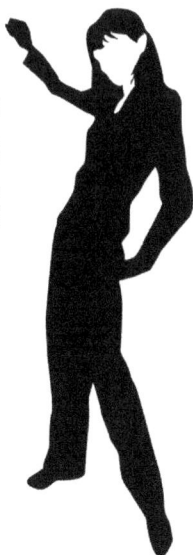

My first job in HIM was as a health data analyst. I was responsible for analyzing emergency room and inpatient records. My job was to make sure that the records were complete and contained no deficiencies (i.e. missing diagnosis, or missing signatures). I had to make sure the record was rerouted to the correct health care professional for correction. My first job was at a great organization where I got a chance to work in many areas on many projects that allowed me to learn and grow as a health information management professional.

KELLI'S
CALL TO ACTION

"Wherever health information is maintained there is an employment opportunity for health information technicians."

What are some companies in your area where health information is maintained?

1) _____

2) _____

3) _____

4)_____

5) _____

Out of the four HIT jobs listed, which job are you most interested in? Why?

_____

_____

_____

_____

_____

_____

_____

_____

_____

What are your salary goals?

1-2 Years _____

3-5 Years _____

10 Years _____

Based on research, are your salary goals achievable?

_____

_____

_____

A HEALTH INFORMATION
TECHNOLOGY
D E G R E E

CAN OPEN THE DOOR TO A VARIETY OF CAREERS

Chapter Highlights

Action Items

- _____

- _____

- _____

- _____

- _____

- _____

- _____

- _____

- _____

- _____

- _____

- _____

Notes

CHAPTER 3
EDUCATION

What you learn in the classroom and at your professional practice experience (PPE) also known as an internship will be essential to your professional career as a Health Information Technician. Throughout your education you will be introduced to your professional organization the American Health Information Management Association (AHIMA), state association, code of ethics and AHIMA's domains, sub domains, and knowledge clusters.

Associate Degree Programs:

A health information technician earns an

associate degree 2 years of formal education in an accredited CAHIIM program from a state, community, or private college. CAHIIM stands for The Commission on Accreditation for Health Informatics & Information Management education which we will discuss further at the end of this chapter. In the students final term or once they complete the program they are eligible to take the Registered Health Information Technician (RHIT) certification exam. In addition, to HIT courses, prerequisite coursework also includes anatomy & physiology, medical terminology, and computer training. Students are also required to complete a PPE in an acute or alternative setting.

Certificate Programs: AHIMA states that coding certificate programs require 6 months to 1 year of education and training. Certification education and training can take place at a public or private school or organization. Certificate programs require students to complete an unpaid PPE. If you want to work in a hospital as a coding professional it is strongly recommended that you will also want to obtain your AS degree. Many employers prefer to see both degree and certificate.

AHIMA states it's important to know the difference between "holding a certificate" and "being certified" in coding. Being certified means you have taken and passed a certification examination. Employers generally wish to hire people who are certified, not just holding a coding certificate of program completion.

Delivery Formats:

When choosing to pursue an associate degree or a certificate program students have the option of completing their education in a traditional campus based program, a hybrid program, or an online program. Below I have listed some of the benefits of each delivery format.

Campus Based Programs: Typically offer classes at a specific time and at a specific location.

- Face to face instruction.
- Access to facilities- School, library, labs.

- Social interaction with peers and teachers.
- Structure with scheduling of courses.

Hybrid Programs: Usually include courses that are campus based & online.

- Course components are online and can be accessed anywhere.
- Regular face to face time with instructor.
- Can keep schedule flexible.
- The learning doesn't stop when you leave the classroom.

Online Programs:

- Can work full time-convenient scheduling.
- Offer flexibility- can study anytime.
- Online education courses bring education right to your home.
- Learn from the comfort of your home.

Accreditation:

The Commission on Accreditation for Health Informatics & Information Management education also known as CAHIIM is an independent accrediting organization that accredits associate, baccalaureate, and masters degree programs. CAHIIM strives to provide the public with effective and consistent quality monitoring of HIM programs through maintenance of accreditation processes. In order to take a certification exam through AHIMA once you complete your AS degree the program you graduate from must be accredited by CAHIIM.

Nothing will work unless you do. ~Maya Angelou

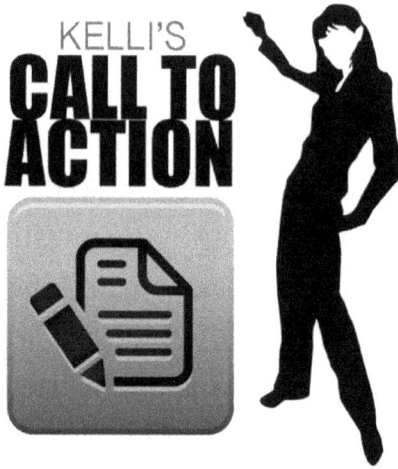

What is your education goal?

_____

How do you believe it will impact your career as a HIT professional?

_____
_____
_____

Which type of delivery format best fits your life? Why?

_____
_____
_____
_____

Chapter Highlights

_____
_____
_____
_____
_____
_____
_____
_____
_____
_____
_____
_____
_____
_____
_____
_____
_____
_____
_____
_____
_____
_____
_____
_____
_____
_____
_____
_____
_____

<u>Action Items</u>

- _____

- _____

- _____

- _____

- _____

- _____

- _____

- _____

- _____

- _____

- _____

- _____

Notes

Notes

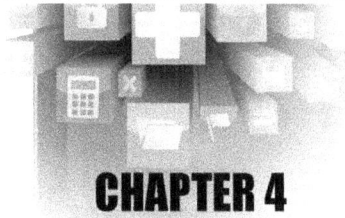

CHAPTER 4
SURVIVING YOUR FIRST YEAR OF SCHOOL

Now that you have decided to pursue a career in Health Information Technology (HIT) and have been accepted into a program you might be wondering what it will take to graduate from the program. Most Health Information Technology programs require that student complete prerequisites before starting their core HIT courses. Prerequisite courses often include Anatomy and Physiology I and Anatomy and Physiology II, Medical Terminology, and a computer course. After your prerequisites course have been successfully completed you are now ready to begin you core HIT courses. During your first year in the HIT program you will take courses that introduce you to the profession, explore laws and regulations pertaining to the HIT profession, and learn how to apply drug classification and medical knowledge to clinical scenarios.

Learning Styles

To make sure you are ready to be the best student you can be I would recommend if you have not identified your learning style I recommend you do. Your learning style means how you learn best. There are many different ways of learning. Each person has a learning style. Below are three common learning styles that people have.

Visual Learner- If you are a visual learner you most likely will do best in an environment that allows you to learn information visually through seeing things. Some suggestions for visual learners would be to take notes, use flash cards, and use a highlighter while studying.

Auditory Learner- If you are an auditory learner you most likely will do best in an environment that allows you to learn by listening. Some suggestions for auditory learners would be to record lectures, watch videos, and repeat what you have learned.

Kinesthetic Learner- If you are a kinesthetic learner then you most likely learns by doing things. Some suggestions for kinesthetic learners would be using flash cards when studying, taking field trips, and studying with others.

To be a successful student and achieve your goal of becoming a HIT student will require you to stay focused on your studies. It is also important that as a student you get the best grades you can get which will show your mastery of the content taught and show your readiness to enter the workforce. In order to make the best grades requires you to make studying a priority. Below I have listed some tips to help you be the most successful student you can be.

Tips to Be a Successful Student:

- **Prioritize**- Obtaining your HIT degree should be your priority. All your decisions should be made around your priority.

- **Preparation**- Come to class prepared with the necessary textbooks required along with paper and a pen or an electronic device to take notes.
- **Participation**- It is important that you participate in class and any other educational activities offered to you through your school and program.
- **Partner** Up- Find a study partner in your program who can help and encourage you.

I would also encourage you to create a plan for graduation and know what courses you will need to take each semester to make sure you are progressing and staying on schedule to graduate on time.

Networking

Networking is the process of getting to know people who can provide you with career guidance or career prospects for you.

Networking also allows you to build professional relationships, connect with someone who could be a mentor to you, or allow you to gain employment at an organization you are interested in working at. So your probably wondering why networking should be important to you as a student. Well, many jobs today do not make it to job recruitment websites. Often many jobs get filled by word of mouth. And even if the job gets advertised job listings tend to draw piles of applicants. It helps to know someone who is already working for the organization you are interested in working. Also, the job you want may not even be advertised, networking can lead to information and job leads. You as a student can start building your network with classmates, professors, friends, and family members. Conferences and networking events are great ways to build your network. You may also want to try building your network through volunteer work, social media, associations, and alumni events. If you have the opportunity to attend a regional or state health information management meeting this is also a great place to network. Don't wait until you need a job to network!

Professional Practice Experience (PPE)

Before you graduate with an associate degree in health information technology you will be required to complete a professional practice experience (PPE). The PPE allows you to get hands on experience in a clinical setting such as a hospital, long term care facility, or doctor's office and apply what you have learned in the classroom. You should consider your PPE a long job interview since where you complete your practicum could become your future employer. The PPE is a course or in some program courses that are include in the course sequence of HIT courses you will be require to complete for your degree. For the PPE instead of going to the classroom you will go to the healthcare site you are assigned to. The number of hours you spend at the site will vary by school. Some schools allow students to spend an entire semester at the healthcare site while others may only require students spend half of the semester at a site. You are not expected to know everything while you are completing your practicum however, it is important to show professionalism by attending your practicum on your scheduled day, arrive on time, stay the entire time you are suppose to, notify the appropriate person in the case of an emergency. Remember you want to make a good first impression. Depending on your school you may be asked to identify practicum sites you are interested in or the program may have sites identified that are available to you.

Tips to Survive Your First Year

- At the beginning of each semester set realistic goals.
- Get to know the expectations of your instructors.
- Get to know your classmates- they make good study partners and potentially add to your network.
- Develop a study schedule each semester that you can stick to.
- Ask for help when you need it. Don't wait until test time of the final exam, to ask questions ask right away!

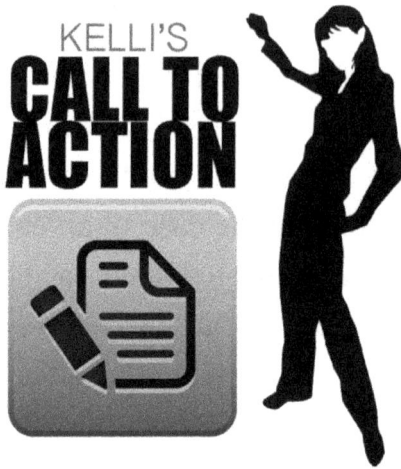

KELLI'S
CALL TO ACTION

What is your preferred learning style?

_____

_____

What are some ways that you can study and better retain the information that you learn?

_____

_____

_____

_____

_____

_____

_____

_____

Build Your Network

Who is your network currently made up of?
How do you think you could add to your professional network?

Chapter Highlights

_____

_____

_____

_____

_____

_____

_____

_____

_____

_____

_____

_____

_____

_____

_____

_____

_____

_____

_____

_____

_____

_____

_____

_____

_____

_____

_____

_____

_____

_____

Action Items

- _____

- _____

- _____

- _____

- _____

- _____

- _____

- _____

- _____

- _____

- _____

- _____

Notes

_____
_____
_____
_____
_____
_____
_____
_____
_____
_____
_____
_____
_____
_____
_____
_____
_____
_____
_____
_____
_____
_____
_____
_____
_____

CHAPTER 5
CERTIFICATION

Certification is one of the most important exams you will take that will lead to you earning a credential. Certification exams test your knowledge, skills, and abilities. Certification is valued by employers and allows you to increase your salary, advance your career, and help you reach your professional goals. Certification lets the world know you are a competent professional. Certification also lets others know that you have taken and passed a national certification exam.

Types of Certification:

There are many certifications an HIT professional may obtain however here I will focus on three in particular. The Registered Health Information Technician (RHIT), Certified Coding Specialist (CCS), and the Certified Professional Coder (CPC).

Students who pursue an associate degree in HIT and are enrolled in a CAHIIM accredited program are able to take the RHIT certification exam whether they are in their final term of study or once they have graduated. HIT professionals who hold an RHIT credential ensure the quality of medical records by verifying their completeness, accuracy, and proper entry into computers systems, use computer application to assemble and analyze patient data for the purpose of improving patient care of controlling costs, and often specialize in coding diagnoses and procedures in patient records. For additional information please visit the American Health Information Management Association website at www.ahima.org Once you are ready to take the RHIT certification exam you will submit your application to the American Health Information Management Association (AHIMA) along with your exam fee which is currently $229 for members of AHIMA and $299 for non-members. Once you have submitted your application and fee you will wait for AHIMA to send you an authorization to test (ATT). You will then be able to schedule your exam through Pearson Vuetesting center. When you receive your ATT it will provide you with a four-month window to schedule your exam.

Some HIT professionals may choose to specialize in coding. Those HIT professionals who specialize in coding often choose to take a certification exam to either earn their CCS-Certified Coding Specialist or their CPC-Certified Professional Coder credential. Those HIT professionals who are generally looking to work in a hospital setting will take the CCS certification exam offered through AHIMA. Certified coding specialists review patient's records and assign numeric codes for each diagnosis and procedures possess expertise in the ICD-9-CM and CPT coding systems, and are knowledgeable about medical terminology, disease processes, and pharmacology. For additional information please visit the American Health Information Management Association website at www.ahima.org AHIMA offers several eligibility routes some of which include having an RHIA, RHIT, or CCS-P credential, or completing a coding training program, or by having a minimum of two years related coding experience. Once you are ready to take the CCS certification exam you will submit your application to AHIMA along with your exam fee which is currently $299 for AHIMA members and $399 for non members. After AHIMA determines your eligibility they will send you an authorization to test (ATT) at which time you will be able to schedule your exam through Pearson Vue testing center. When you receive your ATT it will provide you with a four month window to schedule your exam.

Another coding credential a HIT professional may choose to obtain is a Certified Physician Based Coder credential. The CPC certification exam is offered by The American Academy of Professional Coders. Those HIT professionals who are looking to work in a physician office setting generally pursue the CPC credential. Those who hold a CPC credential are experts in reviewing and assigning accurate medical codes for diagnoses, procedures, and services performed by physicians and other qualified healthcare providers in the office, display proficiency across a wide range of services including evaluation and management, surgery, radiology, pathology, and medicine, have a sound knowledge of medical coding guidelines and regulations, understand how to interpret medical coding and payment policy changes, and knowledge of anatomy and physiology, and medical terminology necessary to code provider diagnosis and services. For additional information please visit the American Academy of Professional Coders website at www.aapc.com The certification requirements for the CPC include having an associate degree (recommended), paying an examination fee of $300 or $260 for AAPC students. CPC exams are proctored by AAPC staff, approved AAPC instructors and local chapter officers.

Don't Delay Certification:

Studies have shown that the longer one waits to take a certification exam after completing their studies the less likely they are to pass. My recommendation would be to take any certification exam as early as you can. Taking a certification right after you have finished your studies increases your chances of retaining what you have learned and being successful on the exam your first attempt. Taking the certification exam as soon as you are eligible will increase your recall of information.

Certification Study Tips:

1. Develop a study schedule of what you will study and when. I would focus first on the areas you feel you are the weakest in. I would also recommend you set aside some time to study with a partner who is preparing to take the same exam as you are. Studying with a partner may provide you with a new way of learning or retaining information.
2. Review materials such as your HIT textbooks, class notes, test, and any examination information provided by

AHIMA or the certifying agency for the exam you wish to take. My recommendation to students is not to sell back or get discard any HIT textbooks until you have passed your certification exam.

3. Attend a certification exam prep workshop. Check with your state association and local college or university in your area to see if they offer a certification exam prep workshop for the exam you are interested in taking. There is usually a fee associated with the workshop however; this will allow you to review material with various people from other schools and cities.

4. Get Clarification. If you are unsure about any aspect of the certification exam such as testing time, what you are allowed to bring with you to the testing site or anything else make sure to contact the certifying organization or testing center as soon as possible.

5. Speak with a recent graduate who has passed the certification exam. This could provide you with helpful insights and motivation.

KELLI'S
CAREER
CHRONICLES

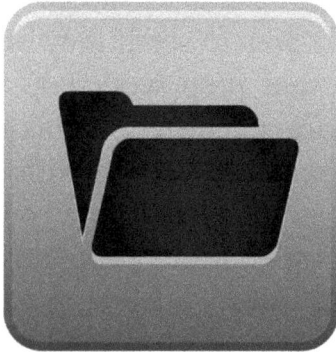

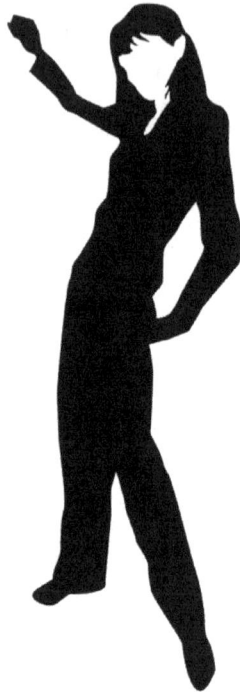

I completed my bachelor's degree in Health Information Management and took and passed the RHIA certification exam. Before I began studying for the exam I set a study schedule that I could stick to. The areas that I was the weakest in I put at the beginning of my study schedule and allotted myself more time to spend on those areas. What I didn't understand I sent time going over that information in my textbooks. I studied up until the day before the examination. I took my RHIA certification exam and passed. My study schedule sure paid off.

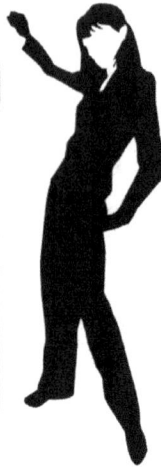

List two ways you will prepare to take the certification exam.

Chapter Highlights

Action Items

- _____

- _____

- _____

- _____

- _____

- _____

- _____

- _____

- _____

- _____

- _____

- _____

Notes

Notes

_____
_____
_____
_____
_____
_____
_____
_____
_____
_____
_____
_____
_____
_____
_____
_____
_____
_____
_____
_____
_____
_____
_____
_____
_____
_____

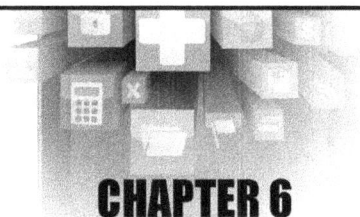

CHAPTER 6
HOW TO LAND YOUR FIRST JOB

Even before graduation approaches you will begin to think about landing your first job as a health information technician professional. You have applied yourself, made good grades and can now see graduation in the near future. Landing your first job as a health information technician professional may seem daunting however; there are some things you can do to make the process less stressful. In this chapter we will explore ways to make your resume stand out, ways to maximize your job search, and interviewing techniques.

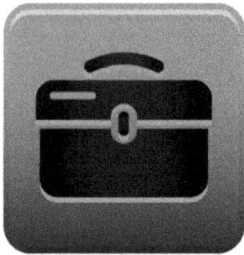

RESUME

Before you apply for your first position you will need to create a resume to market yourself. Your resume will also allow others to know the education, skills, and experience you possess. Before an employer makes a decision of whether to interview you or not they will read your resume. Your resume is competing against hundreds of other resumes so you want to make sure your resume stands out and truly represents you well. Your resume should include your name followed by your educational level, certification you hold, address, professional email at the top of the resume, education you have received or are currently pursuing, jobs that you have had and currently hold with responsibilities you had, any training you have received, any rewards, and references. Once you have created your resume I would recommend you have someone else look over the resume for possible errors or edits that should be made. Remember your resume will make a first impression of you to an employer so you don't want to have any misspelled words. Also, no matter which resume style you go with the ultimate goal is that it looks professional. Recruiters are inundated with resumes so if your resume does not look professional, or information on your resume is hard to find or leaves the recruiter guessing it will get trashed. One resume does not work for all jobs you are applying for. It is important to make sure your resume is tailored to the position you are applying to.

Lastly, you will continue to update your resume your resume will always be changing. Your resume should always reflect any recent education obtained, skills and certifications acquired, and experience you have achieved. Finally, it is important that you have your resume in electronic form and always readily available.

Sample Health Information Technology Resume for New or Recent Graduates

---

Jane Doe, AS, RHIT
123 American Way
Cummings, GA 12345
(123) 456-7890 (cell)
janedoe@domain.com

OBJECTIVE: To obtain a position as a release of information manager with opportunities for professional growth and development.

EDUCATION/CERTIFICATION: American College, December, 2013
AS Degree, Health Information Technology

Registered Health Information Technician, RHIT, December 2013, American Health Information Management Association

EXPERIENCE: Peach Hospital, Cummings, GA
Health Information Technician, August, 2012-present

- Assist physicians with completion of medical records.
- Analyze ER, and outpatient records for deficiencies.
- Process release of information requests.
- Perform other duties as assigned.

Cotton Hospital, Atlanta, GA
Intern, August 2013-December 2013
- Performed audits of reports to determine if any charts were delinquent.
- Processed release of information requests.
- Attended weekly department meetings.
- Participated in department meeting on electronic health record software decision.

PROFESSIONAL MEMBERSHIP: Member of the American Health Information Management Association. August, 2011-present.

COMPUTER SKILLS: Proficient in several computer applications including Word, Excel, Access, and Power Point.

LANGUAGE SKILLS: Read, speak, and write English and Spanish

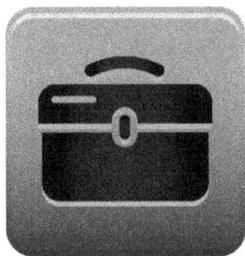

SEARCHING FOR JOBS

Now that you have created your resume you are now ready to begin your job search. The first thing I would suggest as you begin searching for jobs is that you utilize your networking skills discussed in chapter 4 to let people know that you have graduated and are looking for a job. Secondly, exploring the career search of national association websites such as www.ahima.org, www.aapc.org, and your state association website career page will provide you with the latest job postings in your field. Also, if your school has a career service office it may be helpful to see what job postings have been submitted. Make sure to check back often with you instructors to see if any job postings have been submitted to program. Attending career fairs and perusing exhibit halls at conventions are great ways to meet and speak with company representatives who can let you know about opportunities available at their organization and also give you a chance to leave your resume. If there is a particular organization you would like to work for make sure to check their website often. Once you find a position you would like to apply to start out by filling out an application and submitting your resume. Two tips I recommend as you are searching for positions is to keep a folder of the positions that you apply for and to make sure that your resume reflects the position you are applying for. As you are searching for the right position for you and are waiting to hear back from an organization do not get discouraged. Searching for a job can take time. However, don't give up you will receive an employment offer.

Your First Job DREAM Job List

To get the job you really want may take time, but first you have to be clear about what you are looking for. Identify the five companies and entry level positions that would be your DREAM first job. Each month keep an eye on these positions and the requirements that they are looking for. Work on developing those skills and put them in that application's resume.

Company	Position	Skills Required

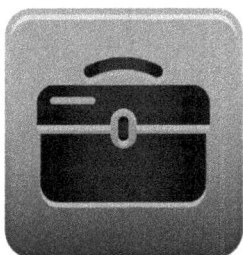

INTERVIEWING

If your resume stands out to a recruiter you may be invited to interview for your desired position. The interview by far is the most important part of the hiring process. If you are invited to interview at a company for a position you must keep in mind that you are competing with many others for the same position. It is important that you make sure you have done your research on the company, your desired position, and are ready to answer any questions you may be asked. During your interview you want to make sure you make a good first impression. The interview begins when you walk in the door. You want to make sure you arrive on time, are polite, and display confidence. As the interviewers begin to ask you questions it is important that you listen carefully and respond to each question clearly and to the best of your knowledge.

Interviewing can be nerve racking however, be sure to relax and just be yourself. You want to give the appearance of looking relaxed and confident. There are many great books and apps that can give you practice at answering common interview questions that you may find helpful to review. I would also encourage you to have some follow up questions written down to ask the interviewers related to any questions you have about the job and also inquire as to when you will hear something regarding their decision on your hire. Lastly, as your interview comes to an end be sure to thank the interviewers for allowing you to interview. Also, be sure to reiterate your interest to work for their organization.

"Some of us are timid. We think we have something to lose, so we don't try for that next hill."

~ Maya Angelou

What is the most challenging part of interviewing for you?

_____

_____

_____

What techniques can you implement to overcome those challenges?

_____

_____

_____

Chapter Highlights

_____

_____

_____

_____

_____

_____

_____

_____

_____

_____

_____

_____

_____

_____

_____

_____

_____

_____

_____

_____

_____

_____

_____

_____

_____

_____

_____

_____

Action Items

- _____

- _____

- _____

- _____

- _____

- _____

- _____

- _____

- _____

- _____

- _____

- _____

Notes

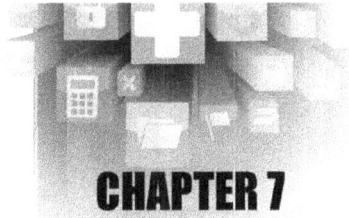

CHAPTER 7
NEVER LET YOUR LEARNING STOP

THE MOST SUCCESSFUL PROFESSIONALS
ARE THOSE THAT OPT-IN TO BE
LIFE-LONG LEARNERS

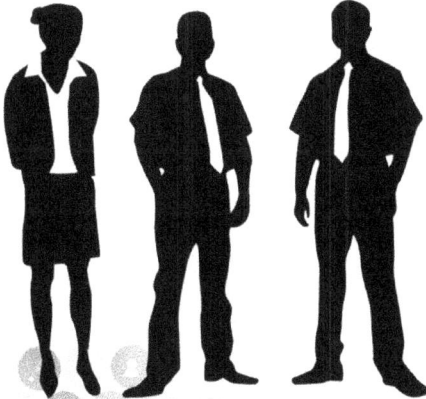

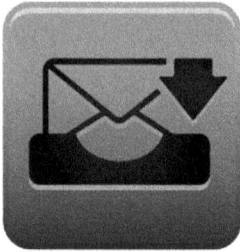

Add to Your Tool Box:

Education and certification does not guarantee you will get a job however; it does make you more marketable. If you are nearing the end of your associate degree or have completed it don't let your learning stop there. I encourage you to either pursue your education onto the baccalaureate level or obtain an additional certification. Increasing your education level or obtaining an additional certification will increase your knowledge in the field, allow you to be considered an expert, increase your earning potential, and increase your employment opportunities.

Certification Maintenance:

Once you obtain your certification in either Health Information Technology, Medical Coding, Cancer Registrar or any other area you will be required to renew your certification with continuing education credits (CEUs) every two years or whatever length of time is deemed by the certifying agency. In order to maintain your certification you will be required to earn continuing education credits and report them during your designated time frame to the certifying agency. Some examples of ways to earn continuing education credits include attending conferences or convention, reading an article, taking a course etc. Once you become certified I encourage you to check with your certifying agency to see what is your reporting time frame for your certification, the costs involved, and ways you can earns CEUs.

Staying Connected:

It is important that after you have earned your degree and certification that you remain connected to a professional association. Belonging to and staying connected with a professional association always you to stay knowledgeable about current events, industry happenings, connected to other professionals, and learn about any industry changes. Some ways in which you can stay connected to your professional association is by subscribing to professional journals whether they be in print or digital form, attending conferences, following the association through social media outlets such as Facebook, Twitter, LinkedIn or by taking continuing education courses or seminars offered through the professional association.

Conclusion:

If you are interested in having a career that allows you to combine your love of science and technology and offers many career opportunities a career in Health Information

Technology may be the right career choice for you. In order to compete in this global economy, people have to be well educated or even consider getting retrained in order to complete for jobs today and jobs that will be available in the future. Jobs in health information are expected to increase by 21% from 2010 to 2020. Don't wait for a job to come to you, get the training and education you need now for the jobs that will be available in the future.

"By asking for the impossible we obtain the best possible."

~Giovanni Niccolini

My Professional Connection Pages

Professional Website _____

Professional Facebook _____

Profession Twitter _____

LinkedIn Account _____

MY LIFE-LONG LEARNER'S
PROFESSIONAL
DEVELOPMENT PLAN

FORMAL EDUCATION

Institution	Program	$

CERTIFICATIONS

Institution	Program	$

CONFERENCES & SEMINARS

Location	Name	$

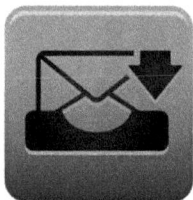

CREATING A CULTURE OF LIFETIME LEARNING

PROFESSIONAL ASSOCIATIONS

PROFESSIONAL JOURNALS & BLOGS

INDUSTRY LEADERS TO FOLLOW	INDUSTRY READING LIST

Chapter Highlights

_____
_____
_____
_____
_____
_____
_____
_____
_____
_____
_____
_____
_____
_____
_____
_____
_____
_____
_____
_____
_____
_____
_____
_____
_____
_____
_____
_____
_____
_____

Action Items

- _____

- _____

- _____

- _____

- _____

- _____

- _____

- _____

- _____

- _____

- _____

- _____

Notes

Appendix

Below you will find helpful additional resources:

1. http://www.ahima.org
The American Health Information Management Association website. Here you can find information about the history of the national association, latest industry developments, career opportunities, can engage with other professionals, and certification options available.

2. http://www.cahiim.org

CAHIIM is an independent accrediting organization that accredits associate, baccalaureate, and masters degree programs. You can browse this website to begin your search of schools in your area that are accredited.

3. http://www.aapc.com

The American Academy of Professional Coders website. Here you can learn about current events, news, and certification opportunities available.

4.http://www.ahimafoundation.org/partners/csa. aspx

This website allows you to search your state association affiliated with American Health Information Management Association.

5.http://hicareers.com/CareerMap/

This website will allow you to search current and emerging health information management careers. The website will also allow you to learn about various job descriptions, job responsibilities, skills needed, and salary information.

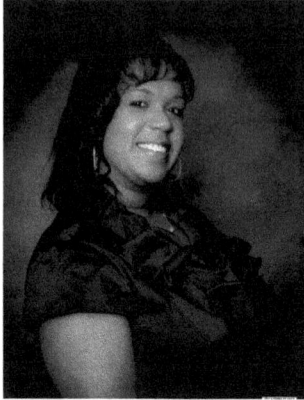

About the Author

Kelli Lewis has been a Health Information Management professional for almost 10 years. Kelli received her bachelor degree in Health Information Management from Florida A&M University and her Masters in Health Informatics from Walden University. She is certified by the American Health Information Management Association as a Registered Health Information Administrator, RHIA. Kelli currently works as a health information management professional and has been teaching health information technology for the last 6 years. She loves to learn about new techie ideas.

Kelli resides in Orlando, FL. She loves to travel, read, and attend musical theater performances.

BOOK
KELLI
LEWIS

FOR YOUR NEXT EVENT

KEYNOTE SPEAKER
WORKSHOP FACILITATOR
GUEST LECTURER

www.kellidlewis.com
E-mail: nandis2013@aol.com

www.ingramcontent.com/pod-product-compliance
Lightning Source LLC
Chambersburg PA
CBHW060622200326
41521CB00007B/850